FUNCTIONAL NEUROLOGICAL DISORDER

TREATING OF FUNCTIONAL NEUROLOGICAL DISORDER MADE EASY

DR. DEAN HIGGINS

Contents

CHAPTER ONE

Beneficial neurological sickness

Useful neurologic ailment — a greater modern-day and broader time period that includes what a few humans call conversion ailment — features apprehensive device (neurological) symptoms that cannot be defined through manner of a neurological illness or distinct medical situation. However, the signs and signs are real and motive large distress or problems functioning.

Signs and symptoms and symptoms and symptoms and signs range, relying on the form of realistic neurologic disorder, and may encompass specific styles. Generally, this disease impacts your motion or your senses, collectively with the capability to walk, swallow, see or pay attention. Signs can variety in severity and can come and go or be persistent. But, you can't deliberately produce or manipulate your signs and symptoms.

The cause of purposeful neurologic ailment is unknown. The state of affairs can be induced via a neurological sickness or via a reaction to strain or mental or bodily trauma, but it's far no longer constantly the case. Useful neurologic ailment is associated with how the mind functions, as opposed to harm to the thoughts's shape (at the side of from a stroke, more than one sclerosis, contamination or damage).

Early prognosis and treatment, particularly

schooling about the circumstance, can help with recovery.

Conversion sickness is a situation wherein a mental fitness trouble disrupts how your brain works. This reasons real, bodily signs and signs that a person can't manipulate. Signs and symptoms and signs can embody seizures, weak point or paralysis, or decreased enter from one or greater senses (sight, sound, and so forth.). This situation is frequently treatable through diverse kinds of treatment.

Functional neurological symptom disorder — better referred to as "conversion sickness" — is a intellectual health circumstance that reasons bodily signs and symptoms and signs and symptoms and signs. The signs and symptoms and symptoms and signs and symptoms stand up due to the fact your mind "converts" the effects of a intellectual fitness hassle into disruptions of your thoughts or stressful tool. The signs are actual however don't in shape up with diagnosed brain-related conditions.

It's critical to take into account that conversion contamination is a real highbrow health circumstance. It's now not faking or interest-seeking out. It isn't genuinely a few component in someone's head or that they've imagined. Even as it's a intellectual health situation, the physical signs and symptoms are though actual. A person with conversion sickness can't control the symptoms and signs in fact via trying or considering it.

What's the difference amongst conversion sickness and somatic symptom disorder?

Professionals company the 2 situations due to the reality there's a outstanding deal of overlap some of the 2, and it's possible to have every on the equal time.

With somatic symptom contamination, you have at the least one symptom that drastically disrupts or interferes together along side your lifestyles. That causes the following:

You spend quite a few time thinking about your symptom(s).

You experience very worried or stressful approximately your symptom(s).

You devote an uncommon quantity of effort and time to the symptom(s) in some manner.

The essential factor characteristic of conversion illness is which you have a thoughts-associated symptom (or a couple of signs and symptoms). Those disruptive signs and symptoms and symptoms hold you from functioning as you may underneath everyday situations. But, you don't have a neurological (mind-associated) situation to offer an reason behind the symptom(s).

Who does it have an impact on?

Conversion ailment can have an impact on human beings sooner or later of their life, which incorporates in the path of youth.

Positive symptoms and symptoms are much more likely at special some time. For example, the common age variety for seizures is amongst a long term 20 and 29, at the same time as the commonplace age variety for particular movement-related signs and signs and symptoms is among 30 and 39.

Conversion sickness is likewise much more likely to take vicinity in girls and people precise girl at begin (DFAB). To be had studies suggests as a minimum twice as many women have conversion disorder in comparison to men or human beings particular male at start (DMAB).

CHAPTER TWO

How does conversion ailment have an effect on my body?

Conversion disease creates disruptions on your thoughts that cause bodily symptoms and signs and symptoms and symptoms. Beneficial MRI — which we ought to professionals see your mind interest — can see the consequences of conversion sickness. People who have conversion sickness normally have much less hobby or uncommon hobby in elements in their mind associated with their signs. Those changes in mind hobby aren't some difficulty someone can fake.

Signs

Signs and symptoms and symptoms and signs and symptoms of useful neurologic sickness can also additionally range, depending at the form of beneficial neurological signs and symptoms and signs and symptoms, and they're splendid enough to cause impairment and warrant clinical assessment. Symptoms and signs and symptoms can have an impact on frame motion and feature and the senses.

Signs and symptoms and signs and symptoms and signs and symptoms which have an impact on frame movement and characteristic might also embody:

Susceptible thing or paralysis

Unusual movement, collectively with tremors or problem walking

Lack of stability

Difficulty swallowing or feeling "a lump within the throat"

Seizures or episodes of shaking and obvious loss of awareness (nonepileptic seizures)

Episodes of unresponsiveness

Signs and symptoms and symptoms which have an impact on the senses can also additionally encompass:

Numbness or lack of the contact sensation

Speech issues, along with the lack of capability to talk or slurred speech

Vision problems, together with double imaginative and prescient or blindness

Being attentive to problems or deafness

Cognitive issues regarding memory and awareness

What motives conversion contamination?

Experts don't understand precisely why conversion ailment takes place. But, they do recognize that it's more likely to appear alongside side sure instances and a few scientific situations.

Common instances visible in human beings with conversion sickness embody:

A data of youngsters abuse.

Having other intellectual fitness conditions, specifically despair or anxiety.

A cutting-edge annoying or annoying occasion.

A cutting-edge day health situation or event performing as a reason for conversion disorder.

Is it contagious?

Conversion ailment isn't contagious, so that you can't get it from others or spread it to others.

Hazard elements

Elements that can increase your risk of sensible neurologic disorder embody:

Having a neurological contamination or sickness, collectively with epilepsy, migraines or a movement infection

Contemporary massive stress or emotional or bodily trauma

Having a intellectual health condition, such as a temper or tension illness, dissociative sickness or positive persona issues

Having a family member with a neurological scenario or signs and symptoms

Having a records of bodily or sexual abuse or forget about in formative years

Ladies may be much more likely than men to increase beneficial neurologic illness.

Complications

A few symptoms of sensible neurologic disease, especially if not dealt with, can result in terrific incapacity and awful remarkable of existence, similar to problems as a result of scientific conditions or disease.

Purposeful neurologic illness can be related to:

Ache

Anxiety issues, which embody panic illness

Melancholy

Insomnia

Fatigue

How is conversion disease diagnosed?

Your healthcare business enterprise can

diagnose conversion disorder the use of a aggregate of bodily and neurological examinations, diagnostic assessments, imaging scans and extra.

Diagnosing conversion disease requires all four of the following:

You have got got one or greater symptoms and signs and symptoms associated with your mind's manipulate over your movement or senses.

Your signs and symptoms and signs aren't constant with diagnosed scientific conditions.

There's no specific purpose to your signs, such as another medical circumstance or intellectual fitness trouble.

The signs or troubles disrupt your life,

mainly your functionality to art work, have relationships, and plenty of others.

What "inconsistent" way with conversion disease

A defining function of conversion sickness is that your signs and signs and symptoms are inconsistent with a identified clinical circumstance. Your healthcare company has to search for methods that your signs and symptoms and signs and symptoms and signs and symptoms aren't normal with one of a kind conditions. That doesn't suggest they don't keep in mind you or your signs and symptoms and signs aren't actual. It technique they want to find out the inconsistency to diagnose conversion ailment.

Finding an inconsistency may not sense like an remarkable component, however in this situation, it's far. Finding inconsistencies amongst your symptoms and symptoms and seemed situations way your healthcare agency can rule out distinctive — and regularly extra-extreme — thoughts-associated problems.

What assessments can be completed to diagnose this case?

The assessments that your corporation recommends rely strongly at the symptoms you've got. In preferred, diagnostic imaging and neurological exams are maximum in all likelihood. Those embody:

Blood exams (the ones can search for some problem from immune device problems to pollutants and poisons, especially notable metals like copper).

Automated tomography (CT) test.

Electroencephalogram (EEG).

Electromyogram.

Evoked potentials test.

Magnetic resonance imaging (MRI).

How is conversion disorder treated, and is there a remedy?

Conversion disease is a intellectual fitness state of affairs that reasons bodily signs and signs and symptoms. Due to that, treating the intellectual health issue with a few shape of psychotherapy (intellectual health remedy) is commonly the number one approach. It's additionally usually the most a fulfillment approach. The maximum common sorts of psychotherapy encompass:

Cognitive behavioral remedy (CBT). That is the most commonplace type of treatment endorsed. Professionals additionally remember it the most in all likelihood to paintings.

Hypnotherapy. This is usually a 2nd preference for styles of remedy. It may be particularly useful on the same time as the signs and symptoms and symptoms of conversion contamination have an impact for your capability to speak or any of your senses.

Company or own family treatment. Shared remedy reviews can assist human beings with conversion ailment. Institution treatment can assist human beings with this example connect to others who have comparable struggles. Family remedy can assist cherished ones apprehend the state of affairs and provide guide.

Other remedies that can assist encompass:

Physical treatment. The symptoms and signs and symptoms of conversion sickness can also moreover start with intellectual fitness, but the physical results are regardless of the reality that real. Physical remedy can help people with conversion disorder get over or adapt to the physical signs and symptoms and signs and symptoms.

Medicine. Even as conversion illness happens

alongside distinct situations, which includes melancholy or anxiety, tablets for those conditions can help conversion illness signs and signs furthermore. That is in particular actual whilst conversion infection motives ache symptoms and signs and symptoms, as antidepressants can regularly truely have an impact on pain stages.

Biofeedback. Biofeedback is an opportunity medication technique that teaches human beings to trade the manner their our our bodies characteristic. It's a mind-body remedy that could enhance your physical and intellectual health. Throughout a biofeedback consultation, your company makes use of monitoring tool and devices to diploma your frame's features. Based totally on feedback from the devices, your company suggests how you may create physiologic modifications. With education and workout, you may learn how to make the ones physical changes without tool.

What am i able to expect if i have conversion disorder?

Conversion ailment is a situation that could have primary results for your life, relying on the signs you've got got. Many human beings who have it experience extreme signs and symptoms and signs and signs that maintain them from on foot or doing sports activities they enjoy.

Many human beings with conversion disorder additionally battle with how they experience about their state of affairs and the manner others cope with them. It's commonplace for people with conversion disease to revel in as although no character believes them or that human beings think they're faking or lying. Often, feeling that no man or woman believes them or accusations of lying — particularly whilst this includes healthcare businesses — hold people from searching out care that could help them.

How prolonged does conversion illness ultimate?

Conversion sickness can very last outstanding lengths of time, counting on severa elements. Those factors consist of whilst it happens on your lifestyles, how excessive it's miles and whether or not or now not you got take care of the situation. An acute case is one in that you've had signs and symptoms and symptoms for under six months. A continual case is one in which signs and signs ultimate for extra than six months.

In some cases, conversion illness is a temporary, short-lived problem. This is most probably in kids but also can show up with adults who get effective care and study their issuer's guidance on dealing with the situation.

For distinctive people, conversion disorder may be a hassle that lasts for years or the relaxation of their life. That is most probably while someone has excessive signs and signs and symptoms, doesn't are searching out care or doesn't comply with through with treatment.

CHAPTER THREE

What's the outlook for conversion ailment?

Conversion sickness isn't a existence-threatening or outright unstable state of affairs. But, it is able to substantially have an effect on your standard highbrow health and properly-being. People with conversion disorder frequently have excessive issues that keep them from operating or taking component in fun sports.

People with conversion disorder are much less probably to have an exquisite final results while the following arise:

Inside the occasion that they postpone looking for health center treatment.

In the event that they do no longer want to simply accept as genuine with they've this situation.

In the event that they don't have an awesome relationship and verbal exchange with their healthcare issuer.

Inside the event that they don't observe the treatment plan their healthcare agency recommends.

The exceptional-case very last results with conversion illness is an entire recovery. As someone improves their highbrow fitness and nicely-being, the disruptions of their mind have to decorate and grow to be a good deal less big until they're lengthy lengthy gone entirely.

How do I cope with myself?

While it is able to feel difficult to recognize how your highbrow health can cause bodily signs and symptoms, it's important to remember that there are various one among a kind conditions in which this happens. Stress, fear, tension and specific horrible emotions can worsen conditions like stomach ulcers, blood pressure and coronary coronary coronary heart troubles.

If you have conversion disease, the satisfactory aspect you could do is art work along with your healthcare corporation and comply with their steering on treatment. Many human beings battle with accepting this prognosis, so you're now not by myself in case you enjoy that manner.

If you conflict with accepting the evaluation, communicate to your healthcare issuer about your issues. Constructing a robust dating at the facet of your provider, wherein you can talk overtly and actually, is one of the most vital subjects you may do to help yourself.

Incredible vital subjects you may and need to do encompass:

Seeing your organisation as endorsed.

Attending and collaborating in therapy periods (which encompass physical treatment, psychotherapy, and so forth.).

Taking your medicinal pills, if any, as prescribed.

How am i able to help a cherished one which has conversion illness?

If you have a loved one that has conversion sickness, your assist may additionally want to make a primary distinction of their recuperation and the very last outcomes of their care.

Here are some beneficial "DOs" and "DON'Ts" to maintain in mind:

DO:

DO validate them. Conversion sickness is a valid clinical circumstance. Humans with it regularly experience like others don't take delivery of as proper with them, a belief that could reason them to resistant to looking for help. Expertise that someone believes them may be a pinnacle encouragement for them to are searching for for care.

DO ask how you could assist. Human beings with conversion ailment can revel in very isolated and by myself. Information that someone wants to assist can make a large difference. You may additionally help through the use of encouraging them to maintain receiving care, specifically in the event that they're suffering.

DO be open to getting to know more approximately their situation and the manner to useful resource them. Your beloved's issuer may additionally want to satisfy with you to speak about the condition. The one which you love or their business enterprise may also moreover ask if you're willing to take part in a treatment session. Remember attending because what you look at need to help you help your beloved better.

DON'T:

DON'T accuse them of faking. Accusing a person of faking the signs and signs and symptoms of conversion sickness — that may be a actual, identified situation — can cause immoderate ache and stress for the only which you love. First-class a informed healthcare business enterprise who has considered all the proof and investigated the signs and symptoms and symptoms and signs and symptoms very well need to ever make that declaration (and healthcare corporations want to most effective say that in the event that they have enough proof to over again it up).

DON'T say it's all of their head. The results of your intellectual health don't just stay in someone's head. Researchers and professionals have tested that intellectual fitness problems have an impact on a person's complete frame and may without problems cause bodily symptoms and signs and symptoms, some of which might be extreme and scary.

DON'T overlook about to take care of your self. Like many particular conditions, conversion disorder can motive strain for the cherished ones of humans with the circumstance. Don't forget about to take care of your private fitness and nicely-being. You can't help someone correctly in case you're struggling to live afloat.

CONCLUSION

Practical neurological symptom sickness, higher referred to as "conversion ailment," is a scenario where a intellectual fitness trouble reasons bodily symptoms and signs and symptoms and signs. This example is actual, and the signs and signs and symptoms and symptoms aren't a few issue someone can manage. Regrettably, many people with this circumstance experience as though others — in particular medical specialists — don't take delivery of as actual with them. This will purpose them to avoid sanatorium remedy that could help them, which typically results in worsening symptoms and signs and signs and symptoms.

When you have conversion sickness or your healthcare organisation tells you they assume it, it's commonplace to revel in scared or involved about what because of this. In case you revel in demanding about this or whether or no longer or not your provider believes you, it's superb to tell your employer about this challenge. Your company's pastime is not to determine you. Their project is to determine what's taking place to you, why it's taking place after which try to address it. If your agency is privy to approximately your concerns and fears, they may be able to try to assist set your mind comfy via paying attention to you and offering guide, advice or solutions.

THE END